# Contents

# Chronotype Diet Cookbook

## Introduction

Whether you stumble into bed before the sun goes up or rise with the roosters, most of us can identify with a specific sleep type or chronotype, even if we've never called it that.

Broken down into four categories, your chronotype shows you when to sleep based on your internal clock. It also gives you insight into all of your main daily activities, such as eating, working, exercising, and socializing.

# CHAPTER ONE

## What are chronotypes?

A chronotype is a person's circadian typology or the individual differences in activity and alertness in the morning and evening.

"Knowing your chronotype may help you understand how your internal clock works and how you can synchronize it with your daily activities and duties to use your time most efficiently," explains Eva Cohen, a certified sleep science coach from Kansas-Sleep.

In particular, Cohen says your chronotype defines your peak productivity times, allowing you to plan your day wisely.

# Chronotypes

## Most research breaks chronotypes into:

Morning type

Evening type

Neither

## Some describe four types, with the names:

Bear

Wolf

Lion

Dolphin

### The bear chronotype

Most people fall under the category of a bear chronotype. This means their sleep and wake cycle goes according to the sun.

Cohen says bear chronotypes wake easily and typically fall asleep with no problem. Productivity seems best before noon, and they're prone to the "post-lunch" dip between 2 p.m. and 4 p.m.

## The wolf chronotype

This chronotype often has trouble waking up in the morning. In fact, Cohen says wolf chronotypes feel more energetic when they wake up at noon, especially since their peak productivity starts at noon and ends about 4 hours later.

Wolf types also get another boost around 6 p.m. and find they can get a lot done while everyone else is done for the day.

## The lion chronotype

Unlike wolves, lion chronotypes like to rise early in the morning. "They may easily wake up before dawn and are at their best up until noon," says Cohen.

Typically, lion types wind down in the evening and end up falling asleep by 9 p.m. or 10 p.m.

## The dolphin chronotype

If you have trouble following any sleep schedule, then you may be a dolphin.

"They often don't get enough sleep due to their sensitivity to different disturbing factors like noise and light," says Cohen.

The good news? They have a peak productivity window from 10 a.m. to 2 p.m., which is a great time to get things done.

## Benefits Of Chronotype

Being able to identify your chronotype can give you insight into your sleep and wake cycles, as well as peak productivity times. Benefits include:

Helps you understand when you fall asleep. Evening chronotypes typically have sleep patterns timed 2 to 3 hours later than morning chronotypes, according to an older study.

Helps you track eating habits. Knowing your chronotype may also help you track eating habits. One review looked at the connection between chronotype, diet, and cardiometabolic health. They found that an evening chronotype, such as wolves, is associated with a lower intake of fruits and vegetables and higher intake of energy drinks, alcoholic, sugary, and caffeinated beverages, as well as higher energy intake from fat.

Helps you understand the connection between sleep-wake time and mental health. Another review found a connection between a number of adverse mental health outcomes, such as depression, for people who have a preference for an evening chronotype, compared to those who identify with a morning chronotype.

## What's my chronotype?

You can find more about your chronotype by taking a quiz:

**The Power of When Quiz**. This one is based on Dr. Breus' book, "The Power of When."

**MEQ Self-Assessment**. The Morningness-Eveningness Questionnaire (MEQ) is another inventory you can take to help determine your sleep type.

**AutoMEQ.** You can also use the automated version.

Your chronotype depends on several factors, including genetics, environment, age, and sex, according to one study.

Researchers also reported that older adults identify more with a morning chronotype, while teens and younger adults tend to fit the evening type.

When it comes to gender differences, they found that males are more inclined to be associated with an evening chronotype, which may be due to endocrine factors.

## How to apply this information

Identifying and understanding your chronotype and sleep cycles can help you maximize your wake time and sleep better at night.

Dr. Nate Watson, SleepScore Advisor and co-director of the University of Washington Medicine Sleep Center, says when it comes to sleep and chronotypes, the majority of people are neither morning or evening type.

In other words, they fall into the "neither" category. This means their sleep shouldn't be affected.

However, he does point out that people who are evening types will desire a later bedtime and rise time than morning types.

While chronotypes are mostly fixed, Watson does say that exposure to light in the morning may help an evening type fall asleep earlier, and exposure to light in the evening may help morning types go to sleep later.

Additionally, Watson says evening type chronotypes may do best with careers that don't require an early start time in the morning or careers with flexibility regarding when the work gets done. And morning type chronotypes would do best working traditional hours.

Sleep is best if it occurs predominantly at night, regardless of chronotype," says Watson. "I recommend both chronotypes (morning and night) listen to their bodies and go to bed when they feel tired and arise when they feel rested."

# How to Calculate When You Should Go to Sleep

How much sleep did you get last night? What about the night before? How much sleep do you actually need?

Keeping track of your sleep schedule may not be a top priority, but getting enough sleep is critical to your health in many ways.

You may not realize it, but the amount of sleep you get can affect everything from your weight and metabolism to your brain function and mood.

For many people, wake-up time is a constant.

What time you go to sleep, however, tends to vary depending on your social life, work schedule, family obligations, the newest show streaming on Netflix, or simply when you start to feel tired.

But if you know what time you have to get up, and you know you need a specific amount of sleep to function at your best, you just need to figure out what time to go to bed.

In this article, we'll help you understand how to calculate the best time to go to bed based on your wake-up time and natural sleep cycles.

We'll also take a closer look at how your sleep cycles work and how sleep can affect your health.

## How much sleep do you need?

How much sleep you need changes throughout your lifetime. An infant may need up to 17 hours of sleep each day, while an older adult may get by on just 7 hours of sleep a night.

But an age-based guideline is strictly that — a suggestion based on research of how much sleep you may need for optimal health as your body's needs change.

According to the American Academy of Pediatrics and the CDC, these are the general sleep guidelines for different age groups:

## Sleep guidelines

Birth to 3 months: 14 to 17 hours

4 to 11 months: 12 to 16 hours

1 to 2 years: 11 to 14 hours

3 to 5 years: 10 to 13 hours

6 to 12 years: 9 to 12 hours

13 to 18 years: 8 to 10 hours

18 to 64 years: 7 to 9 hours

65 years and older: 7 to 8 hours

Everyone's sleep needs are different, even within the same age group.

Some people may need at least 9 hours of sleep a night to feel well rested, while others in the same age group may find that 7 hours of sleep is just right for them.

The biggest question is how you feel when you get various amounts of sleep. Here's what to keep in mind when evaluating your own sleep needs:

The biggest question is how you feel when you get various amounts of sleep. Here's what to keep in mind when evaluating your own sleep needs:

## Do you feel rested after 7 hours of sleep, or do you need at least 8 or 9?

Are you having any daytime drowsiness?

Are you reliant on caffeine to get you going throughout the day?

If you sleep with someone else, have they noticed you having any sleeping issues?

Signs you're not getting enough sleep

Sleep deprivation is a real thing for some, especially as work and life stress builds up. Getting too little sleep can affect many of your body's systems and restorative functions.

**You may also be getting too little sleep due to:**

Insomnia

Obstructive sleep apnea

Chronic pain

Other conditions

**Some signs you may not be getting enough sleep include:**

You're drowsy during the day

You're more irritable or moody

You're less productive and focused

Your appetite has increased

Your judgement and decision-making isn't what it usually is

Your skin is affected (dark undereye circles, dull complexion, droopy corners of the mouth)

A 2020 sleep study showed that sleep deprivation doubled the odds of making placekeeping errors and tripled the number of lapses in attention.

Sleep and mental health are closely connected, with sleep disorders contributing to depression and anxiety. Sleep is one of the most important factors in our overall health.

## Sleep calculator

**Bedtimes are based on:**

Your wake-up time

Completing five or six 90-minute sleep cycles

Allowing 15 minutes to fall asleep

**Wake-up time Bedtime:**

7.5 hours of sleep

**(5 cycles) Bedtime:**

9 hours of sleep

(6 cycles)

4 a.m. 8:15 p.m. 6:45 p.m.

4:15 a.m. 8:30 p.m. 7 p.m.

4:30 a.m. 8:45 p.m. 7:15 p.m.

4:45 a.m. 9 p.m. 7:30 p.m.

5 a.m. 9:15 p.m. 7:45 p.m.

5:15 a.m. 9:30 p.m. 8 p.m.

5:30 a.m. 9:45 p.m. 8:15 p.m.

5:45 a.m. 10 p.m. 8:30 p.m.

6 a.m. 10:15 p.m. 8:45 p.m.

6:15 a.m. 10:30 p.m. 9 p.m.

6:30 a.m. 10:45 p.m. 9:15 p.m.

6:45 a.m. 11 p.m. 9:30 p.m.

7 a.m. 11:15 p.m. 9:45 p.m.

7:15 a.m. 11:30 p.m. 10 p.m.

7:30 a.m. 11:45 p.m. 10:15 p.m.

7:45 a.m. 12 p.m. 10:30 p.m.

8 a.m. 12:15 a.m. 10:45 p.m.

8:15 a.m. 12:30 a.m. 11 p.m.

8:30 a.m. 12:45 a.m. 11:15 p.m.

8:45 a.m. 1 a.m. 11:30 p.m.

9 a.m. 1:15 a.m. 11:45 p.m.

## What are the stages of sleep?

When you fall asleep, your brain and body go through several cycles of sleep. Each cycle includes four distinct stages.

The first three stages are part of non-rapid eye movement (NREM) sleep.

The last stage is rapid eye movement (REM) sleep.

The NREM stages used to be classified as stages 1, 2, 3, 4, and REM. Now it's generally classified in this way:

**N1 (formerly stage 1):** This is the first stage of sleep and the period between being awake and falling asleep.

**N2 (formerly stage 2):** The onset of sleep begins at this stage as you become unaware of your surroundings. Your body temperature drops slightly, and your breathing and heart rate become regular.

**N3 (formerly stages 3 and 4):** This is the deepest and most restorative sleep stage during which breathing slows, blood pressure drops, muscles relax, hormones are released, healing occurs, and your body becomes re-energized.

**REM:** This is the final stage in the sleep cycle. It takes up about 25 percent of your sleep cycle. This is when your brain is most active and dreams occur. During this stage, your eyes move back and forth rapidly under your eyelids. REM sleep helps boost your mental and physical performance when you wake up.

It takes, on average, about 90 minutes to go through each cycle. If you can complete five cycles a night, you'd get 7.5 hours of sleep a night. Six full cycle's are about 9 hours of sleep.

Ideally, you want to wake up at the end of a sleep cycle instead of in the middle of it. You usually feel more refreshed and energized if you wake up at the end of a sleep cycle.

## Why is sleep important?

Sleep is crucial for many reasons. A good night's sleep:

Regulates the release of hormones that control your appetite, metabolism, growth, and healing

Boosts brain function, concentration, focus, and productivity

Reduces your risk for heart disease and stroke

Helps with weight management

Maintains your immune system

Lowers your risk for chronic health conditions, such as diabetes and high blood pressure

Improves athletic performance, reaction time, and speed

May lower your risk of depression

# Tips for better sleep

To improve your sleep health, consider the following tips.

## During the day

Exercise regularly, but try to schedule your workouts at least a few hours before you go to sleep. Exercising too close to bedtime may lead to interrupted sleep.

Increase your exposure to sunlight or bright lights during the day. This can help maintain your body's circadian rhythms, which affect your sleep-wake cycle.

Try not to take long naps, especially late in the afternoon.

Try to wake up at the same time each day.

## Before bed

Limit alcohol, caffeine, and nicotine in the evening. These substances have the potential to interrupt your sleep or make it difficult to fall asleep.

Switch off electronics at least 30 minutes before bedtime. The light from these devices can stimulate your brain and make it harder to fall asleep.

Get into the habit of a relaxing routine before bedtime, like taking a warm bath or listening to soothing music.

Turn down the lights shortly before bedtime to help your brain understand that it's time to sleep.

Turn down the thermostat in your bedroom. 65°F (18.3°C) is an ideal sleeping temperature.

**In bed**

Avoid looking at screens like the TV, your laptop, or phone once you're in bed.

Read a book or listen to white noise to help you relax once you're in bed.

Close your eyes, relax your muscles, and focus on steady breathing.

If you're unable to fall asleep, get out of bed and move to another room. Read a book or listen to music until you start feeling tired, then go back to bed.

If you're aiming for 7 to 9 hours of sleep each night, a sleep calculator can help you figure out what time to go to bed based on your wake-up time.

Ideally, you'll want to wake up at the end of your sleep cycle, which is when you're most likely to feel the most rested.

A good night's sleep is essential to good health. If you're having trouble falling asleep or staying asleep, consider talking to your doctor. They can help determine if there's an underlying cause.

# CHAPTER TWO

## CHRONOTYPE RECIPES

### Roast Chicken With Arugula Puree

**Ingredients**

Chicken file

Arugula

Dill

Small zucchini

Sea salt

Spices per your taste

**Preparation**

Chop chicken meat into slices, rub with your favorite spices and place in baking bag. Before the end of baking, cut the bag and let meat get nice golden color. Put a little water in the pan, add washed arugula and zucchini peeled and chopped into cubes. Briefly cook and mash into blender to get puree. Add little olive oil, salt, chopped dill and if you like little garlic

## Onion And Mushrooms Stuffed Chicken

### Ingredients

Chicken fillet

Onion

Mushrooms

Asparagus

Rocket salad

Lemon

Sea salt

Olive oil

## Preparation

Cut the chicken fillet longitudinally and tenderize using meat mallet. Chop onion into cubes and mushrooms into slices. Fry onion with vegetables on little oil until soften and spice with salt and pepper. Stuff chicken meat with fried onion and mushrooms. Attach with toothpick to prevent stuffing leak out and grill. Also, grill asparagus. Wash rocket salad and season with salt, olive oil and lemon. Decorate and enjoy.

## Perch With Vegetables

### Ingredients

Perch fish

Spinach

Kale

Sea salt

Lemon

Garlic

Fresh or dried parsley

## Preparation

Adjust the quantities to the number of persons and appetite. Clean and wash the fish. Rub it with salt, place chopped garlic inside, wrap in a foil and bake with little water in the oven. Bake about half an hour, then remove foil and let fish get nice golden color. Serve with green non-starchy vegetables.

## Spicy Chicken Kebabs

### Ingredients

800 g minced chicken fillet

1 onion

2 garlic cloves

1 egg white

Pinch of baking soda

Sea salt

Pepper

1 teaspoon paprika

2 tablespoons hot roasted red pepper sauce

**Preparation**

Mix minced chicken meat with hot roasted red pepper sauce, chopped onion and garlic and egg white. Add baking soda, salt, pepper and paprika. Mix well all and form kebabs. Fry them on allowed oil for frying or on a grill pan and serve with lettuce.

## Chicken In The Greek Way

**Ingredients**

1 chicken fillet

Juice of 1 lemon

2 garlic cloves

1/2 teaspoon black pepper

1 teaspoon sea salt

1/3 teaspoon paprika

Little olive oil

## Preparation

Cut the chicken fillet into three steaks, tenderize little using meat mallet. Mix olive oil, lemon juice, chopped garlic, salt, pepper and paprika. Place the meat in some dip dish and pour prepared marinade over it. Leave in the fridge for at least one hour. Bake prepared chicken steaks on a grill or grill pan and serve with arugula salad, or other salad per your taste.

# Egg Whites Omelet With Mushrooms

## Ingredients

100 g mushrooms

4 egg whites

1/2 green belly pepper

1 handful baby spinach

Sea salt, pepper

Allowed oil for frying

## Preparation

Chop the mushrooms into slices, green belly pepper into rings and peel baby spinach. Heat little allowed oil in a frying pan, add prepared mushrooms and fry them constantly stirring until softened and until the excess liquid evaporates. Then add green belly pepper and briefly fry them, and then add spinach. Whisk the egg whites slightly with little salt and pour over vegetables. Don't stir any more, just cover the pan and fry on moderate temperature until the underside of the omelet gets golden color. Then using spatula, turn the omelet upside down carefully and fry the other side as well.

## Hake Stuffed Peppers

### Ingredients

6 green belly peppers

1 large onion

500 g hake fillet

1 bunch of chard

1/2 young zucchini

2 egg whites

Sea salt, pepper

Allowed oil for frying

## Preparation

Scoop out belly peppers and clean of the seeds and stalks. Peel onion and chop into cubes, as well as hake fillet. Wash chard, remove stalks and chop into stripes, and zucchini completely with the skin into rings. Fry onion on little oil, add hake and continue frying constantly stirring until fish get nice golden color. Add chopped chard and stir. Add salt and pepper and remove from the heat. Add egg whites into chilled mixture and stuff peppers with that. Close peppers with zucchini rings. Arrange in greased baking dish and pour with little water. Cover with foil and bake in preheated oven on 200 degrees about 40 minutes. Then remove foil and continue baking until peppers get nice golden color

## Chicken With Herbs

### Ingredients

1 whole chicken (app. 2 kg)

1 bunch of dill

1 bunch of parsley

1 bunch of thyme

2 cm ginger root

Grape seed oil

1 onion

1 fennel

1 lemon

Sea salt, pepper

## Preparation

Wash dill, parsley and thyme and chop into larger pieces. Gradually prepare marinade: mix grated ginger and lemon zest with lemon juice and grape seed oil. Add little sea salt and pepper and stir. Wash the chicken, lift the skin with a knife and separate from the meat. Coat the space between meat and skin with the prepared marinade, then arrange the twigs of parsley, dill and thyme. The rest of marinade rub on the outside of the chicken and the inside of the chicken stuff with chopped onion, fennel and the rest of herbs. Place chicken into baking dish covered with baking paper. Cover with foil and bake in preheated oven on 200 degrees about 80 minutes. Then remove foil and continue baking until skin get nice golden color.

## Lamb's Lettuce Salad

### Ingredients

80 g lamb's lettuce (corn salad)

2 large cucumbers

3 tablespoons olive oil

1/2 lemon

300 g chicken fillet

Sea salt, pepper

**Preparation**

Wash lamb's lettuce and spice per taste. Arrange on two plates and sprinkle with lemon juice and olive oil. Chop one cucumber completely with green skin into circles, while peel other one and hollow out balls using some little sharp spoon. Cook chicken meat into salted water, leave to cool and then chop into slices. Arrange meat and cucumber over prepared lamb's lettuce, try and spice per your taste.


## Chicken Kebabs With Kohlrabi

**Ingredients**

400 g chicken fillet

1 tablespoon Dijon mustard

1 teaspoon curry

2 large kohlrabi

Oregano

Allowed oil for frying

Sea salt, pepper

## Preparation

Cut the chicken lengthwise into strips. Put the meat into bowl, add mustard, 2 tablespoons of oil, curry and oregano. Also add salt and pepper per taste, mix well and leave in the fridge to rest for at least 60 minutes. Arrange marinated meat on wooden skewers. Peel kohlrabi and chop into thin slices, and spice per your taste. Cover baking dish with baking paper, sprinkle with oil and arrange kohlrabi on it. Bake in preheated oven on 200 degrees until get nice golden color. Fry chicken kebabs on heated oil to get nice golden color on both sides and serve with baked kohlrabi and cucumber salad.

## Sardine Stuffed Peppers

## Ingredients

2 green belly peppers

1 sardine can

1 handful baby spinach

2 egg whites

100 ml mineral water

Sea salt, pepper

Allowed oil for frying

**Preparation**

Cut green peppers completely with petiole lengthwise into halves and clean from the seeds. Wash baby spinach and chop into stripes, take out sardines from the can and drain from the oil. Stuff halves of green peppers with spinach and sardines. Separately whisk the egg white with mineral water and little salt. Pour prepared mixture over stuffed peppers. Arrange peppers on a baking paper sprinkled with oil and bake in preheated oven on 200 degrees until get nice golden color.

# Chicken And Zucchini Roll

## Ingredients

500 g chicken fillet

2 zucchini

1 leek

2 green belly peppers

Little allowed oil

1/2 bunch of parsley

Sea salt

## Preparation

Cut the tops from zucchini and then completely with the bark chop into thin slices. Cut the chicken meat into steaks, tenderize using meat mallet and spice with little salt. Chop leek into rings and peppers into sticks and gently fry them on little oil until soften. Take transparent foil and cut into appropriate size. Arrange zucchini slices over foil so that they overlap at the ends, then place chicken over the zucchini and then fried peppers with the leek over the meat. Then carefully roll with the help of foil. Cook prepared roll in boiling water for 15 minutes. Leave to cool, remove foil and cut into slices.

## Cauliflower Steaks

### Ingredients

1 large cauliflower

Sea salt, pepper

Grape seed oil

3 – 4 tomatoes

1 small onion

2 garlic cloves

1/2 leek

## Preparation

Separate the cauliflower from the roots and outer leaves, and use a sharp knife to cut the head into steaks, making sure they don't fall apart. Spice steaks with salt and pepper from both sides. Heat the oil in a frying pan, arrange "steaks" and fry them 3 – 4 minutes from one side, then turn them carefully to fry from other side. Separately prepare salsa: blanch tomatoes, then peel them and finely chop, add chopped onion, leek and garlic. Srpinkle with little oil and serve with prepared cauliflower steaks.

## Mackerel With Kale

### Ingredients

1/2 leek

1/2 kale

Sea salt, pepper

Fresh parsley

Mackerel can

**Preparation**

Finely chop leek and fry on little allowed oil and little water. Then add chopped kale and fry together until soften. Add salt, pepper and chopped parsley. Serve with mackerel from the can and sprinkle with lemon juice.

## Mediterranean Bread

**Ingredients**

200 g spelt flour

200 g rye flour

2 eggs

1 teaspoon sea salt

1 baking powder

150 ml mineral water

150 ml sour milk

50 ml olive oil

100 g sunflower seeds

2 – 3 sprigs rosemary

10 leaves of basil

**Preparation**

Whisk the eggs, add mineral water mixed with sour milk, oil, flours, salt, baking powder and fresh herbs (rosemary and basil). Knead the dough and leave to rest for half an hour. Form the loaf, place on a baking paper. Bake on 200 degrees about 30 minutes.

## Pizza Triangles

**Ingredients**

Buckwheat phyllo dough

Little lukewarm water

Roasted red pepper sauce or tomato sauce

Ham

Feta cheese

Oregano per taste

**Preparation**

Take one sheet of buckwheat dough, sprinkle with lukewarm water, place little cheese, roasted red pepper sauce and ham. Then fold from one side, then from from other side and roll to get triangle. You can place some seeds on top and thin slice of butter. Bake for about 20 minutes at 220 degrees to get nice golden color.

## Salty Cake

**Ingredients**

2 cups spelt flour

1 cup oat flour

1 egg

1/2 cup allowed oil

1 teaspoon sea salt

250 g cottage cheese (crumbled or grated)

5 - 6 green olives (chopped)

Chopped green part of spring onion

Few slices of ham or chicken breasts

1/2 baking powder

1 chopped red pepper

Little mineral water

**Preparation**

Mix all dry ingredients, add chopped vegetables, cheese, egg and finally oil and mineral water to get compact that isn't too much hard, it should be soggy mixture. Pour into greased baking dish or covered with baking paper and bake on 180 degrees about 30 minutes.

Due to combination of cheese and egg, this is complicated dish and should be consumed once in 14 day. If you want to enjoy in it more often replace whole egg with egg white.

## Buckwheat Pie With Meat

### Ingredients

500 g buckwheat phyllo dough

1/2 kg minced beef meat

3 onions

Olive oil

Sea salt

Pepper

### Preparation

Finely chop onion and fry it on oil with meat and spices. Grease baking dish with oil, then place three sheets of phyllo dough (each greased well with oil and mineral water), then put a layer of meat and so on for as long as you have meat and phyllo sheets. At the end put three layers of phyllo. Cut the pie into cubes, grease well with oil and mineral water and bake on 230 degrees about half an hour or until get a nice golden color.

## Stuffed Buns

### Ingredients

4 buns

4 sprigs of spring onion (green part)

1 clove of garlic

200 g mushrooms

2 eggs

Sea salt

Allowed oil for frying

## Preparation

Cut chrono buns at the top, keep covers on the side and scoop out the middle and crumble it. Chop green parts of spring onion into cubes, mushrooms into slices and mash garlic. Pour little oil in the pan, add green part of the spring onion and mushrooms. Fry occasionally stirring until vegetables soften and until excess fluid boils. Remove from the heat and cool. Add mashed garlic, crumbled middle of the buns and two eggs. Spice with salt and mix well. Stuff prepared buns with that mixture, arrange in a baking dish covered with baking paper. Bake in prehated oven on 200 degrees about 20 minutes.

In the same way, you can stuff other chrono pastry.

## Salad With Chickpeas

### Ingredients

150 g chickpeas

1 lettuce

2 carrots

1/2 red cabbage

150 g young cheese

Little olive oil

Lemon juice

Mixture of dried herbs

Sea salt

**Preparation**

Soak chickpeas into water previous day and
leave overnight. In the morning pour out
that water, add new and cook until softened
or about 40 minutes. Remove from the heat
and leave covered to swell. Chop lettuce and
red cabbage into strips, coarsely grate
carrots and chop onion into rings. Place in a
bowl lettuce, cabbage and carrot, spice per
taste, add onion and sprinkle all with lemon
juice. Then add chickpeas drained of water
and young cheese and sprinkle all with olive
oil.

# Hummus With Avocado

## Ingredients

200 g cooked chickpeas

1 ripe avocado

2 tablespoons tahini paste

3 garlic cloves

Juice of 1/2 lemon

Sea salt, pepper

Little olive oil

## Preparation

Cut, slice, peel and pit avocado. Put cooked chickpeas into blender, add avocado chopped into cubes, tahini paste, lemon juice and mashed garlic. Mix gradually adding olive oil until get compact mixture. Before the end of mixing add salt and pepper per taste. Pour prepared hummus into sterilized glass jar, cover it and keep in the fridge until serving. Use it within 2 to 3 days.

## Pie With Nettle And Young Cheese

**Ingredients**

500 g buckwheat phyllo dough

1 piece of young cheese

1 handful blanched and chopped nettle

2 egg whites

2 tablespoons olive oil

Little sea salt

**Preparation**

Mix all ingredients. Take three sheets of phyllo dough, grease each with little mineral water and oil, then place prepared mixture on third sheet and arrange in a baking dish. Then take other three sheets, repeat procedure until you have ingredients.

Instead of this kind of ordering you can wrap the pie as a snail. In that case bake in round baking dish, otherwise use rectangular baking dish to arrange pie. Bake on 200 degrees for about 15 minutes, then more 15 minutes on 150 degrees.

## Colorful Scrambled Eggs

### Ingredients

1/2 yellow pepper

1/2 zucchini

3 eggs

Pinch of sea salt

1/2 tomato

Chopped parsley

Pork fat for frying

## Preparation

On a little pork fat fry yellow pepper chopped into cubes, then add zucchini also chopped into cubes and fry until vegetables get nice golden color. Then add whisked eggs with salt and when eggs start frying add tomato also chopped into cubes and chopped parsley. Just stir and that's it. Serve with chrono bread or some chrono pastry and some fresh salad.


## Pizza With Arugula Pesto

### Ingredients

**For the dough:**

480 g spelt flour + 40 g for sprinkling

1/4 teaspoon sea salt

1 baking powder

320 ml water + allowed oil for greasing

**For the stuffing:**

50 g arugula

3 garlic cloves

4 tablespoons grape seeds oil

3 red peppers

150 g bacon

250 g mozzarella

**Preparation**

Mix spelt flour, sea salt and baking powder. Gradually pour lukewarm water and knead soft dough. Form the ball and leave to rest for five minutes, then knead again for seven minutes to become elastic. Divide into four parts and form each in a ball. Place them on a floured dishcloth, cover with wet dishcloth and leave to rest for 60 minutes. Wash arugula and mix with chopped garlic and grape seed oil and mix in a blender. Chop red pepper into circles, bacon into stripes and mozzarella into thin slices. Take one ball and stretch it into disc with your palms.

Turn the round baking tray (25 cm diameter) upside down and place the pizza on it and form it so that the edge of the dough remains a little thicker. Grease with arugula pesto, arrange red peppers, bacon and mozzarella over it. Repeat the procedure with the remaining balls of dough. Heat the oven on maximum temperature and bake until get nice golden color.

## Zucchini And Chard Galette (Waffles)

### Ingredients

1 young zucchini

50 ml oil

1 bunch of chard

3 garlic cloves

2 eggs

Little sea salt

1 baking powder

150 g spelt flour

Allowed oil for frying

## Preparation

Peel zucchini and grade it, but don't drain from excess fluid. Wash chard and blanche in salted water to soften. Drain from excess water and finely chop. Mix in a bowl grated zucchini, blanched chard, mashed garlic, eggs and little sea salt and stir well. Add mixture of spelt flour and baking powder and mix well to get compact mixture. Grease waffle maker, pour one ladle of mixture in it, cover and bake until get nice golden color.

## Nice Salmon Spread

### Ingredients

200 g marinated salmon fillet

150 g mascarpone cheese

1 organic lemon

1/2 bunch of dill

1 teaspoon grated horseradish

2 tablespoons olive oil

Pepper

**Preparation**

Wash lemon and make zest and juice. Wash dill, drain and finely chop. Also chop salmon fillets. Mix in a bowl mascarpone cheese, pinch of sea salt, lemon zest and lemon juice. Add grated horseradish, chopped salmon and dill. Mix well to get nice, compact mixture. Chop some chrono bread or chrono pastry and richly spread prepared mixture over it. Sprinkle with pepper and enjoy combining it with some fresh salad.

# Rustic Pie With Spinach

## Ingredients

300 g spelt flour

50 g barley flour

1 tablespoon psyllium

1 teaspoon sea salt

1 teaspoon baking powder

60 g butter or pork fat

200 ml water

200 ml sour milk

300 g cottage cheese

2 garlic cloves

100 g baby spinach

## Preparation

Mix in a bowl spelt and barley flour, then add salt, baking powder, psyllium and butter. Pour lukewarm water and knead the dough. Cover it with kitchen cloth and leave to rest for ten minutes. In separate bowl whisk the egg using fork, then take the small part of it and leave for coating, while the rest add to prepared dough as well as sour milk. Knead once again in soft dough and leave to rest for 20 minutes. In a meantime wash spinach and finely chop garlic. Mix in a bowl spinach, garlic and cottage cheese, add little salt per taste. Transfer the dough to floured working surface and stretch using rolling pin into thin circle. Cover round baking tray with baking paper, transfer dough into it. Place prepared spinach filling into the middle and align using spatula, and wrinkle the ends of the dough and fold toward the center. Coat folded ends with lukewarm water and the whiped egg you saved, sprinkle with little flour to get rustic look. Bake in preheated oven on 200 degrees about 40 minutes.


## Salad From Jar

## Ingredients

1 small cucumber

50 g cherry tomatoes

1 small red belly pepper

1 young carrot

1 sprig of spring onion

Few leaves of chicory

1 leaf of fresh crystal lettuce

Few sprig of fresh parsley leaves

Juice of 1/2 lemon

1 garlic clove

2 tablespoons olive oil

Sea salt

Basil

## Preparation

Wash cucumber and chop completely with green skin into thin circles, chop cherry tomatoes in halves, red pepper into stripes, carrot and spring onion into circles and chicory and crystal lettuce into larger pieces. Mash garlic and mix with olive oil, lemon juice, basil and chopped parsley. Sterilize a glass jar and pour prepared marinade on the bottom, then arrange cucumber, cherry tomatoes, pepper, crystal lettuce, chicory and spring onion. Close the jar and just before eating, turn it upside down and shake it until the marinade is evenly spilled.

## Omelet Rolls With Chard

### Ingredients

3 chard leaves

4 eggs

Sea salt

Allowed oil for frying

## Preparation

Wash chard leaves, remove stalks and chop into stripes. Separate egg whites from egg yolks and whisk egg yolks with little salt. In other bowl foamy whisk egg white with little salt. Add chopped chard in a egg yolk mixture and stir well. Then add whisked egg whites and gently stir. Grease baking pan and heat it, then pour one half of prepared mixture in it. Fry until get golden color on bottom side, then gently turn using spatula and keep frying other side. On the same way fry one more omelet. Roll omelets, cut into large slices and string on cocktail skewers and serve with some nice ham.

## Scones With Cheese

### Ingredients

200 g spelt flour

150 g rye flour

1 teaspoon baking powder

1 teaspoon sea salt

25 g butter

75 g young cheese

1 egg

2 dl sour milk

Sesame for sprinkling

**Preparation**

Mix in a bowl spelt and rye flour, then add salt, baking powder, butter and cheese. In other bowl whisk the egg using fork, then separate little mixture for coating, while the rest add to first mixture. Also add sour milk and knead soft dough. Form ball and leave to rest for 20 minutes. Then transfer dough on floured working surface and stretch using rolling pin into circle. Transfer to a baking dish covered with baking paper and cut crosswise into 8 triangles. Coat with egg and sprinkle with sesame. Bake in preheated oven on 200 degrees about 25 minutes until get golden color.

# Fine Salmon Spread

## Ingredients

200 g marinated salmon fillets

150 g mascarpone cheese

1 lemon

1/2 bunch of dill

1 teaspoon grated horseradish

2 tablespoon olive oil

Sea salt

## Preparation

Use one lemon to make zest and juice. Finely chop salmon fillets, as well as dill. Mix in a bowl mascarpone cheese, salt, lemon zest and 2 tablespoons of lemon juice. Add grated horseradish, chopped salmon and dill and mix to get compact mixture. Coat some chrono bread or pastry with this delicious spread and enjoy perfect breakfast.

# Aromatic Salmon Fillets

## Ingredients

500 g salmon fillets

1 bunch of dill

1 lime

2 sprigs of spring onion

1 small onion

50 ml grape seed oil

Sea salt, pepper

## Preparation

Chop salmon fillets into four pieces. Finely chop dill, and use lime to get zest and juice. Chop spring onion into rings and onion into cubes. Mix in a bowl chopped onion, dill, grape seed oil, zest and lime juice. Add pinch of salt and pepper. Grease baking dish, arrange salmon fillets in it and pour prepared marinade over each piece of fish.

Bake in preheated oven on 200 degrees about 30 minutes.

## Red/Green Muffins

**Ingredients**

1 cup spelt flour

1/2 cup rye flour

1/2 buckwheat flour

1/2 baking powder

1 teaspoon sea salt

1 cup sour milk

1/2 cup olive oil

1 egg white

2 tablespoons roasted red pepper sauce or tomato sauce

1 handful chopped spinach

**Preparation**

Mix all ingredients, pour into silicone molds for muffins and bake on 200 degrees about 20 to 30 minutes.

## Stuffed Waffles (Stuffed Galette)

**Ingredients**

2 cups allowed flour per taste

1/3 cup pork fat

Sea salt

Egg white

Baking powder

Little lukewarm water

Sesame seeds

Sunflower seeds

Flax seeds

## Preparation

Knead the compact dough hard enough to make balls, not too large. Place that balls on a baking paper and press with some dish which have round bottom. Then on every second stretched dough place some filling per your taste: roasted red pepper sauce, ham, cheese... and fold with another round dough. You can leave them covered overnight and bake them in the morning using waffle iron, or make all in the morning and then bake.

## Mix Buckwheat Pie

### Ingredients

1/2 kg buckwheat flour

1 baking powder

1 teaspoon sea salt

200 g cottage cheese

2 leek

1 zucchini

4 dl mineral water

6 tablespoons olive oil

## Preparation

Chop leek and zucchini and fry on little olive oil and water. Mix flour with baking powder and salt. Add water and oil, then add crumbled cheese and fried and chilled leek and onion. Stir all once again and pour mixture into greased baking dish or covered with baking paper. Sprinkle with sesame. Bake about 35 minutes on 220 degrees.

## Fast Pie With Ham

### Ingredients

400 g buckwheat phyllo

200 g ham

2 sour cream

200 g Emmental cheese

Olive oil

**Preparation**

Grease one sheet of phyllo with olive oil, place second over it, place one tablespoon of mixture you prepared from chopped ham, sour cream and cheese. Form by folding into triangles which you'll arrange in a greased baking dish. Bake in preheated oven on 200 degrees about half an hour.

## Buckwheat Snail Pie

**Ingredients**

8 sheets of buckwheat phyllo dough (maybe more, less ... it depends how much snails you want to make)

500 g cottage cheese

1 egg or just egg white

100 ml water

Few slice of butter

**Preparation**

Crumble cheese with the fork, add egg, whisk and salt to taste. First sprinkle each sheet of phyllo dough with water. Put little prepared filling (about 1-2 tablespoons on one sheet) and roll it diagonally, then form a shape of snail. Arrange prepared snails on a baking dish covered with baking paper and put slice of butter on each. Bake in preheated oven on 200 degrees about half an hour until get nice golden color.

## Gnocchi With Pesto, Broccoli And Pine Nuts

**Ingredients**

500 g chrono gnocchi

500 g broccoli

100 g pine nuts

2 – 3 tablespoons pesto

Little butter

Sea salt, pepper, basil, nutmeg

Parmesan slices

### Preparation

Cook gnocchi as directed. Separately cook broccoli. Melt butter in a pan, add cooked broccoli, little pesto, salt, pepper, basil and nutmeg. Pour prepared mixture over the gnocchi and sprinkle with Parmesan and roasted pine nuts.

## Cottage Pie with Leafy Green Vegetables

### Ingredients

1 kg spelt flour

1/2 kg cottage cheese

1/2 leafy green vegetables

4 eggs

100 ml olive oil

1/2 butter

Baking powder

Sea salt

**Preparation**

Mix flour with baking powder, add oil and enough water to knead dough. Leave it to rest for 1/2 hour at warm place. Stretch the dough. Prepare stuffing from crumbled cheese, chopped leafy green vegetables, eggs and butter. Add salt if necessary and arrange over the dough. Fold the dough and bake in the oven on 200 degrees about 40 minutes.

## Cauliflower In The Dough

**Ingredients**

600 g cauliflower

4 eggs

3 tablespoons flour (spelt, rye, buckwheat)

150 g butter

2 tablespoons grated Parmesan

1 tablespoon chrono bread crumbs

Parsley

Sea salt, white pepper

## Preparation

Foamly whisk egg whites. Divide cauliflower into florets and blanch it. Whisk butter, add egg yolks, flour and finely chopped parsley. Add salt and pepper. Stir the mixture gradually adding whisked egg whites. Finaly add blanched cauliflower. Pour mixture in a baking dish greased with butter and sprinkled with chrono bread crumbs. Bake in the oven until get nice golden color. Cut into slices and sprinkle with Parmesan.

# Scrambled Eggs With Vegetables And Seeds

## Ingredients

Small piece of bacon

1/4 red belly pepper

Few mushrooms

Sesame seeds

Flax seeds

2 eggs

Chopped parsley

## Preparation

Add chopped bacon in a heated frying pan, fry for few minutes, add chopped red belly pepper – few minutes, then add chopped mushrooms and fry a little bit longer because mushrooms have a lot of water in itself. When the water evaporate, add sesame and flax, stir 2 to 3 times and finely add whisked eggs. Fry for two minutes and serve with chrono bread and some spread like hummus, roasted red pepper sauce or with some fresh salad.

## Conclusion

Getting a good night's sleep is essential to both your physical and mental health.

Being able to identify and understand how your chronotype affects your sleep and wake time can help you maximize productivity, gain insight into your health, and learn new ways to increase the quality of your sleep.

Though we all need sleep, we don't all follow the same sleep schedule or have the same sleep needs. Paying attention to your sleep habits and cycles and learning more about your chronotype can help you get better control of your sleep schedule and make it easier to get healthy rest at night (and wake up feeling refreshed in the morning).

Printed in Dunstable, United Kingdom